INTERVIEWING PROCEDURES

INTERVIEWING PROCEDURES

A Manual for Survey Interviewers

by

J. Stacy Adams

Chapel Hill

The University of North Carolina Press

Foreword

This manual is an attempt to strike a balance between the cookbook variety of manual and the treatment of interviewing usually found in texts of sociology and social psychology. As a result, the manual not only presents basic general principles and procedures of interviewing, but also gives the rationale behind them. The author hopes that the interviewer using this manual will learn both the "how" and "why" of interviewing techniques.

An attempt has been made to write a manual which would be useful to all survey interviewers. However, some material, especially the section on sampling, applies particularly to procedures which have been used by the Survey Operations Unit, University of North Carolina. To enhance the general utility of the manual, details and examples which are necessarily specific to a given situation have been kept to a minimum, and recommended practices have been presented as principles. In general, the principles are guides, allowing some freedom in their application, rather than rigid statements of step-by-step methods. Accompanying the statement of each principle is a discussion of its rationale and of its application. To facilitate the use of the manual, a glossary and an index have been provided, and footnotes have generally been omitted. The manual has also been printed in a format small enough to permit it to be carried easily in the field.

In planning and writing this manual the author has benefited from the ideas and advice of many persons. Individuals who have contributed greatly, directly and indirectly, are Nancy Campbell, John Monroe, and John W. Thibaut. An expression of appreciation is also due J. Mayone Stycos for permission to use material on probing contained in his book, *Family and Fertility in Puerto Rico: A Study of the Lower Income Group*. Very helpful also have been the chapter on interviewing by Eleanor and Nathan Maccoby in the *Handbook of Social Psychology*,

Herbert Hyman's *Interviewing in Social Research,* and the University of Michigan's Survey Research Center *Manual for Interviewers.* Charline Hardison is thanked for typing the manual. Finally, the Institute of Statistics and the Institute for Research in Social Science, University of North Carolina, are thanked for making the writing of this manual possible.

Contents

CONTENTS

CHAPTER I

The Interview Survey: Introduction

A. *Brief History of Surveys*

It is probable that surveys have, in a very broad sense, existed as long as Man himself, for it is not too much to assume that men have always had to consider, if not to respect, the wishes, opinions, needs, and behavior of other men with whom they were in contact. Man's early "surveys" may have been no more than fortuitous observations, but they were nevertheless surveys of their social environment. Early written records indicate that rulers kept a close touch on the public pulse, even if their "interviewers" were little better than spies.

Planned, systematic surveys are of comparatively recent origin, however, and as one might guess one of the first was government sponsored. This was the United States Census of 1790, which collected information on family size, number of freeholders, number of slaves, and so forth, in order to determine how many representatives each state would have in Congress in accordance with a provision of the Constitution. Since then the United States and other governments have greatly increased the use of surveys in the fields of housing, labor, consumer finances, health, and morale. Some of these surveys have been of the census type, enumerating the population completely, but most have been sample surveys, in which a few persons were selected to represent the population. One of the first sample surveys was the social survey of five industrial cities in Great Britain conducted by Arthur Bowley in 1912-14. Compared with today's complex sampling procedures, Bowley's method was simple: he picked every twentieth house systematically from a list.

The surveys best known to the public are probably the public opinion polls of voting intentions. One of the first was done by the Raleigh, North Carolina, *Star* in 1824, when it sent its reporters to cover political meetings throughout the state and to find out who was likely to win the forthcoming election. In the latter part of the nineteenth century and early in the twentieth century the Boston *Globe,* the New York *Herald,* the Des Moines *Register and Tribune,* the *Farm Journal,* and the *Literary Digest* began their own polls. The most famous of these were perhaps the *Literary Digest* presidential straw polls which began in 1916 when the candidates were Hughes and Wilson. The *Digest* correctly predicted the outcome of this election as well as subsequent ones until 1936, when it predicted the election of Landon over Roosevelt—a decidedly erroneous prophecy. It was at about this time that other famous polls made their start: the Gallup Poll, the *Fortune* magazine survey, and the Crossley Poll.

Somewhat before the *Literary Digest* fiasco, market and audience surveys came on the scene. In 1921 James McK. Cattell, a famous psychologist, organized the Psychological Corporation, which initiated brand preference studies. Five years later the General Foods Corporation established a panel of housewives to test its products, and, a few years after, the General Motors Corporation organized a consumer research department. Thereafter, especially after World War II, independent market and consumer research organizations proliferated, as did similar organizations within large corporations. The growth of audience and mass media surveys closely followed that of market surveys. Indeed, the growth of both resulted partly from the popularization of radio and the associated development of radio advertising. "Hooperatings" of radio programs began in 1934 under the direction of C. E. Hooper. The major networks did surveys of large samples of the population. To facilitate the measurement of program preferences the "audimeter" was invented by A. C. Nielsen and the Lazarsfeld-Stanton "program analyzer" was devised to analyze the content of programs. With the advent of television after World War II a new impetus was given to audience studies, and a large number of professional and trade journals now regularly publish survey findings.

In the past twenty years surveys have become a major tool of industry, government, and social science. Today sample surveys are used in arriving at important decisions—decisions which, to a greater or lesser extent, affect almost everyone. The fare on television is largely influenced by public opinion surveys. The package design of a certain brand of cigarettes or the silhouette of a new automobile model reflect public expressions obtained in surveys. Farm and crop supports by the government and regulations governing the Federal Reserve System are in part predicated on the findings of interviews. The appearance of a new product on the grocery store shelf may be a direct result of a careful marketing survey. The amount of space devoted to "hard" news in a chain of newspapers is very likely in part based upon a mass media survey. The content of broadcasts to Iron Curtain countries is guided by careful interviews with refugees. Important sociological, psychological, and political studies conducted by major universities make use of the survey technique. The distribution and kind of health services made available by local, state, and federal authorities are often predicated on the findings of sample surveys.

Although they have not always been used wisely or conducted with scientific detachment, surveys have nevertheless contributed to progress in a democratic society. They have, in fact, been the basis for important economic, political, and social decisions.

B. *The Interview Survey as a Communication Process*

Although personal interview surveys date back to at least the fourth quarter of the nineteenth century, there has been frequent misunderstanding of the processes and objectives of surveys even among practitioners. As is often the case when attempting to understand something, it is well to make oneself as naive as possible and to ask apparently simple questions. One such question is: *What is the purpose of a survey?* It is to obtain information, or more precisely, to reduce one's uncertainty. A survey is conducted to collect information in order that there be less uncertainty about an existing state of affairs, a decision to be made at some future date, or the occurrence of a future event. For example, a survey may be done to reduce the Department of Labor's uncertainty about the income of skilled machine operators, or to reduce uncertainty about a decision to market a new home appliance, or to reduce uncertainty about the outcome of a political campaign.

The next question one may ask is: *What is the medium through which information is sought?* It is usually language (verbal questions). A researcher who uses survey data seeks to reduce his uncertainty about something by obtaining information collected by an interviewer who asks questions. *What is the medium through which information is given?* It is again language, or some equivalent form of symbolic response. That is, a respondent answers an interviewer's questions verbally or, equivalently, by placing a check mark next to a written statement.

It is apparent from the answers to the above three questions that the information-seeking relationship between interviewer (who is the researcher's agent) and respondent is essentially one of *communication*. Furthermore, even though it is the interviewer who is seeking information, the communication is a two-way system, from interviewer to respondent and, in reverse, from respondent to interviewer. If the interviewer will remember that he and the individuals he interviews are communicating with each other his task should be greatly facilitated, for many of the principles of interviewing are in reality principles of communication.

The role of the interviewer is all-important. Upon the functions which he performs a survey stands or falls. This is not to say that his role is the only important one; the study director, the sampling statistician, the analysts, the coders all have equally important roles. If any one fails in his functions the survey will be more or less of a failure. The interviewer and other members of a survey team are interdependent parts; the goal can be achieved only if each functions properly.

CHAPTER II

The Phases of an Interview Survey

The interview survey usually consists of several broad phases, which, although not independent of each other, may be considered separately. The phases are: statement of the research problem, instrument construction and pretesting, sampling, interviewing, processing and analyzing the data, and reporting the results. Even though a particular person may be concerned with one or two phases only, it is desirable that he have some knowledge and appreciation of all aspects of a survey. It is the purpose of this chapter to provide this knowledge and to develop this appreciation by describing each phase briefly.

A. *Statement of the Research Problem*

The statement of the research problem is logically and necessarily the first step in any well-planned survey for the decisions made during later phases are contingent upon it. It is concerned with answering the question, *What is it we are to find out?* The answer given to the question must be as specific as possible in order that the problem may be translated into operational terms for use in subsequent phases, such as the questionnaire and sample design.

An example will illustrate simply what is done during this phase of the survey. A tobacco manufacturer desires to determine how much people smoke. This is the over-all problem, but it is stated far too generally to be practical. What is the referent for "people" in this case? How is "smoking" to be defined? What is meant by "how much"? These questions must be answered carefully. "People," in this instance, may be all the employees of the tobacco company; "smoking" may refer to the consumption of cigarette, cigar, and pipe tobacco by burning and oral aspiration; and "how much" may refer to the average daily consumption of cigarette, cigar, and pipe tobacco in grams. With these specifications the *universe to be surveyed, the subject* of the survey, and the *unit of measurement* to be used are known. In turn, decisions about *sampling, instrument construction,* and *interviewing procedures* can be made.

B. *Instrument Construction and Pretesting*

In the context of this manual the term *instrument* refers to the devices with which specified events and objects are measured, and the term *questionnaire* refers to a collection of instruments. Generally the instruments are questions to be asked of respondents, but they may also be a set of scales to weigh cigarette butts and tobacco residues, or a photometer to measure illumination, or a tape to measure the dimensions of a corn field, depending on what the survey problem is. Other devices employed in surveys are card-sorting, paired comparisons of objects, projective tests, sentence completion tests, and story-telling about pictures.

The two core problems in the design of instruments are *validity* and *reliability*. Validity has reference to whether the instrument measures what it is intended to measure. Frequently validity is assumed, for no external criteria exist whereby it can be assessed. On the other hand, it must be said, in fairness, that the assumption of validity is often tenable because of the nature of the questions and the answers to them. For example, the response, "the twelfth; I graduated from high school," to the question, "What is the highest grade you completed in school?" indicates the question has some validity, especially if other data obtained are congruent with high school education. This is only face validity, however, and it would be desirable to have better evidence. For example, in the illustration above, it would be well to have the school records of the individual to ascertain validity.

The reliability of an instrument in survey work has to do with whether the same answers are obtained to the same questions on different occasions. As with validity, reliability is frequently assumed, rather than demonstrated. An instrument is said to be perfectly reliable to the extent that it gives the same measurement under identical conditions. This perfection is never attainable, however, and reliability is therefore usually given as a fraction or proportion of a theoretical maximum. Questions, just as physical instruments, are reliable only within specific limits of error. The problem facing the survey researcher is therefore one of reducing error to a minimum.

Question-wording has a major role in establishing the validity and reliability of survey instruments. Unless wording is carefully done accuracy will suffer. How carefully words have in fact been chosen is usually indicated by the results of *pretesting*—that is, trying questions out on people. Many pretests are usually conducted and revisions made after each before the questions are judged sufficiently valid and reliable to be used in a survey. The validity and reliability of questions is thereafter in the hands of the interviewer. If he does not use them as instructed the answers obtained are unreliable and of unknown validity.

C. *Sampling*

Only rarely are all members of a specified universe (e.g., adult U.S. citizens, employees of the Acme Tobacco Company, farm implement dealers in Middle Western states) interviewed in the course of a survey. To do so would be uneconomical. Instead it is the practice to estimate the characteristics (e.g., political opinions, smoking habits, income, recreation habits) of the universe under consideration from the characteristics of a few appropriately selected individuals who are representative of the universe. The selection of these individuals is all-important, and the ability to make generalizations from them to the universe is predicated upon *appropriate sampling*.

What is appropriate sampling? It is not a procedure, for there are many ways of selecting samples which are representative of the universe. Rather, it is a set of requirements imposed upon the means of selecting *units* from a specified universe (e.g., occupied dwelling units, individuals, farms). The primary requirement is that the probability or chance of selecting a particular unit be known. The most popularly known *probability* sample is the *random* sample, in which all units of the universe have an equal, and therefore known, chance of being selected in the sample. The well-publicized selection procedure used by draft boards in World War II is an example of simple random sampling: if a thousand names were in the mixing cage, the first name drawn had one chance in one thousand of being selected. Other types of sampling are more complex, but are nevertheless based on the known-probability principle. The procedure described in Chapter IV is an example.

When the requirements of appropriate sampling are met it is possible to estimate universe characteristics from sample characteristics within specific limits of accuracy. These limits depend upon the number of units in the sample, the variability of the characteristic in the universe, and, to a lesser extent, upon the ratio of the number of units in the sample to the number in the universe.

One further important point should be made about sampling. Although a sample is designed and selected in the office of the survey researcher, the final identification of units is often made by the interviewer according to prescribed procedures. It is therefore essential that the sampling specifications be met accurately by the interviewer.

D. *Interviewing*

Since interviewing is the subject of this manual little will be said about it here. It is the process of collecting information from respondents by an interviewer with the aid of a questionnaire. In practice this does not completely define the job of an interviewer, however, for he must also do some sampling and related tasks.

A key concept in interviewing is *communication*. The interviewer must be able to communicate without distorting the questions designed by the researcher. He must establish an atmosphere which will maximize the communicativeness of the respondent; that is, he must communicate an atmosphere of permissiveness. Finally, he must be able to communicate information obtained from a respondent to the researcher. How this can be done is the subject of the next chapters.

E. *Processing and Analyzing the Data*

After survey data have been collected they must be analyzed, interpreted, and reported. It must be evident that in most surveys it would be impractical, if not impossible, for the analyst to deal directly with the questionnaires. It is therefore necessary to reduce questionnaire data, frequently including long, complex answers, to some manageable form. The over-all process of so doing is referred to as *coding* and consists of translating questionnaire answers into a compact set of symbols, usually numbers. These numbers may then be transferred to punched cards, and the data originally contained on bulky questionnaires may thus be compactly stored.

When the analyst desires to tabulate certain data from the punched cards he has the cards placed in a tabulator (or other machine) which will give him the desired information in printed code form. He may then retranslate the code symbols into conventional linguistic form, that is, into words, and proceed with his analysis and interpretation.

F. *Reporting the Results*

The report of findings brings the survey to an end at the point where it originated: the problem. If the statement of the problem was accurate and each phase following it was conducted diligently the report should answer or suggest a solution to the problem.

Each major phase of an interview survey has been described briefly, as if it were independent of other phases. This is, of course, not the case: all phases are related. The statement of the research problem determines what universe will be sampled, what questions will be asked, what interviewing procedures will be used, and so on. *How* questions are asked is also related to the characteristics of the individuals who will be sampled. For example, interviewing Southern sharecroppers requires a somewhat different questionnaire and approach than interviewing farmers in the Middle West area on the same subject. The sample design also in part determines *what* questions are asked. For instance, in some cases the household may be the ultimate sampling unit and an adult may be asked to answer questions about the whole household, whereas in other cases the individual may be the ultimate sampling unit and he answers questions about his own behavior. Thus, research problem, sample, and questionnaire are intimately interrelated. In turn, the processing and analysis of data are determined by the preceding phases, but it is also true that the careful researcher will plan data processing and analysis at the very beginning of a survey in order to decide what data to collect, how to collect them, and from how many respondents to collect them. The initial and final phases are therefore mutually interdependent. Because all phases are so closely related, it is obvious that failure to accomplish any one phase properly will result in the failure of the total project to meet its objectives.

In making final decisions about the research problem, the sample, the number of individuals to be interviewed, the interviewing procedures, and data processing, cost enters as a major consideration. Answers to the research problem are obtained with a specific degree of accuracy at a stated cost. Cost and accuracy are directly related, for greater accuracy increases cost. If there is an upper limit on cost the limits of accuracy must be governed by it or the research objective revised. Conversely, if cost is not a factor, as much accuracy as desired is theoretically possible. Where both cost and accuracy have specified limits, the research problem must be formulated to permit adherence to the cost and accuracy factors.

CHAPTER III

Interviewing

This chapter represents an attempt to set forth a number of principles which, when applied, will result in sound interviewing. The principles have been deliberately kept broad whenever possible so as to serve as guides rather than as restrictive chains. The reasons underlying most principles have been explained in detail to enable the interviewer to understand and use them flexibly and effectively. Although several examples of the application of the principles have been given, their use has been limited in order not to give the impression that the principles are applicable only to the cases illustrated. Quite the contrary is true: it is intended that the principles cover a wide range of situations. In some sense, then, the principles represent a "philosophy" of interviewing rather than unchangeable, inflexible rules.

Although the principles presented in this chapter are fundamental to sound interviewing, they may be modified or countermanded in the case of some surveys for rather specific purposes. Whenever this is the case the interviewer will receive specific instructions to that effect along with other special instructions pertaining to the survey. Each survey differs in detail, and close attention must always be given to the specific instructions which accompany it. In some instances these instructions or "survey specifications" may be as long as this manual.

A. *Introducing the Survey and Establishing Rapport*

The success of each interview depends considerably on the ability of the interviewer to create a friendly, permissive atmosphere of mutual trust and confidence when the respondent is first contacted. There is no one best way of establishing this rapport, for the best way of doing this with one respondent will be inadequate with another. People differ in socio-economic status, character, health, and experience with interviewers and salesmen, and they have different expectations of "pollsters." These differences must be taken into account, and exactly how this is done is dependent on how sensitively the interviewer perceives these differences and can adapt the interview situation to them. Needless to say, establishing rapport cannot be done instantaneously; it takes place throughout the course of the interview. The first impression made on the respondent is very important, however, for it "sets" the respondent to perceive the interviewer and the survey in a manner which may be either beneficial or detrimental to the purpose of the survey. In general, the respondent should be made to perceive that the interviewer is permissive and is doing an important job. Conversely, he should never be made to perceive that, so far as the interviewer or survey sponsors are concerned, there are right or wrong, good or bad, acceptable or unacceptable, or better or worse answers to anything asked during the interview. The respondent should feel, for instance, that being Republican or Democrat, buying brand X or Y, driving a Chevrolet or Cadillac, going to church or not, liking or disliking his neighbors, rooting for the Yankees or the Red Sox, viewing Steve Allen or Ed Sullivan, loving or hating children, or being well or poorly educated are equally acceptable.

How can this atmosphere of permissiveness be established? It must first be said that the desired atmosphere can be established only to a greater or lesser degree. Some respondents encountered are so defensive in their personality structure that no amount of effort on the interviewer's part will lead them to believe anything they say is all right. As a result their answers to questions, rather than being "true," may be modified to suit a false perception they have of the interviewer, brought about by peculiar personality needs. On the other hand, almost ideal rapport can be established with other respondents. There is no way of knowing beforehand how desirable an atmosphere can be created, and it is therefore necessary to follow certain principles which are likely to bring about rapport. As applies to most principles, they should be used intelligently and adaptively in accordance with situational needs—the nature of the survey, the characteristics of the respondent, the place of interview, and so forth.

1. *The interviewer must introduce himself and state the purpose of his call.* Aside from being courteous, such an introduction serves to dispel immediately any suspicion that the interviewer is a salesman. This is important, for if the interviewer is perceived as a salesman a prompt refusal to be interviewed may follow, or, if the respondent agrees to be interviewed his responses may be biased. This would be especially serious if the subject of the survey dealt with consumer goods or other

products. In order to avoid the possible appearance of a salesman, it is good practice not to carry a briefcase or other suggestive paraphernalia. Only the papers needed should be carried to the door, and these should be arranged neatly so as to preclude awkward fumbling when interviewing begins.

The introduction should cover the following four important points:

—a. *Who is conducting the survey.* Introductory statements should indicate that the organization by whom the interviewer is employed is reliable. This should overcome possible suspicions that a hard or soft "sell" is in the offing, or that a government, credit, or collection agency is making an investigation.

—b. *The subject and purpose of the survey.* The subject and purpose of the survey should be stated rather broadly, for if given in too much detail answers to subsequent questions may be suggested. For example, it definitely would be better to say that the purpose was to study "people's TV viewing preferences" than to say that the purpose was "to find out if people like Steve Allen." In some cases it may be desirable to hide the purpose of the survey in the introductory remarks, because knowledge of the purpose might bias answers or result in lack of cooperation. An example might be a study of race relations. In such cases a purpose other than the real one must nevertheless be given, and the interviewer should be given appropriate instructions by his supervisor.

Merely stating that the interviewer is doing a "survey" has been found insufficient and troublesome, because many respondents in the past have had a "sales pitch" introduced under the guise of a "survey." For example, two interviewers recently reported lack of cooperation because the respondents had invited a "surveyer" in, who then promptly tried to sell them a set of encyclopedias. A general statement of the purpose of the survey and emphasis of the fact that the respondent's *ideas* are what is wanted will usually overcome this type of difficulty.

—c. *How the respondent happened to be chosen.* Respondents are very frequently curious, even suspicious, about how they, in particular, were chosen to be interviewed. Unless they are given a satisfactory answer they may think that the interviewer has an ulterior motive and, as a result, give biased answers. An explanation which will usually satisfy a respondent is that he was chosen by chance by a process of calling at every fifth house or so in the neighborhood. If warranted, more details may be given. Showing a map or list to the respondent is often convincing evidence of the selection procedure.

—d. *The interview is confidential.* Although it sometimes does not matter whether a respondent is told that the answers obtained in the interview are confidential, it is safer to point this out explicitly. In no case should the point be given much emphasis, however, unless the respondent raises the issue. Emphasis on the confidential aspects of the survey arouses suspicion in many people and makes others excessively self-conscious, for a "confidential" interview might imply that something in the interview might cause embarrassment if revealed.

2. *The interviewer must make the respondent feel that the interview situation is permissive.* This principle has already been alluded to, but deserves reiteration. It is the objective of every survey, no matter what its subject, to obtain "true" answers. But many people will modify the "true" answers if they perceive that some other answer will be better liked (or less well liked) or make more sense (or less sense). Hence, permissiveness must be established; how well and quickly will vary from interview to interview. It is probable that a few questions and answers will be required, since the only way to convey permissiveness is by proof—that is, by the interviewer's neutrally accepting and recording whatever the respondent says. It is in part to establish permissiveness that many surveys begin with a few questions which do not require probing or checking.

In creating an atmosphere of permissiveness, it is important not only that the interviewer show no sign of disapproval but also that he give no indications of approval. This is rather difficult and requires practice in the use of a variety of neutral signs such as "uh-huh," "I've got that," a simple nod, "yes, I see." By the same token the interviewer should not give the impression of too much friendliness; he should not establish too much rapport. To do so might imply approval of certain things reported by the respondent.

There is one exception—not to answers given to questions, but to how the respondent generally behaves during the interview. If a respondent is cooperative, approval of this should be indicated. Conversely, if a respondent is unruly, careless, or uncooperative, a mild but straightforward sign of disapproval should be made. An interview may otherwise quickly become worthless. Whether approving or disapproving, the interviewer should remain business-like at all times.

3. *The interviewer must make the respondent feel that the survey is important.* People are generally more likely to cooperate if the survey in

which they are requested to participate is shown to be important, though it need not be directly important to the respondent. The statement that a survey is of direct importance to every respondent is often so patently unlikely that it is insulting. It is therefore best, when possible, to state frankly the purpose of the survey, why and to whom it is important. For example, respondents will readily accept as important a hat manufacturer's interest in people's color preferences even though they may never wear, or intend to wear a hat. On this basis they would probably cooperate willingly, yet would refuse to be interviewed if they were told that their answers would someday determine what color of hat they would wear.

4. *The interviewer must make the respondent feel that his answers are important.* Respondents often find it difficult to understand why it is important for them, in particular, to answer the survey questions, especially when they have been told that they were chosen by chance. They should be told that chance selection is the only way to guarantee an unbiased cross-section of people, and that since they are part of the cross-section the interview with them is very important.

A related point which respondents should, but do not always, understand is that their *own* true answers to questions are important, no matter how unrepresentative they might be. Respondents who, for example, have extreme opinions or are otherwise atypical frequently say, "You don't want to interview me. I'm very different from most people around here and my answers would mess up your survey." This is quite wrong, of course; atypical answers are just as important to survey researchers as are "average" ones. If this point is understood, conveying the idea of permissiveness should be facilitated and the respondent's motivation to cooperate should be increased.

5. *The interviewer's appearance must be neutral.* An interviewer's physical appearance, including clothing, accessories, and make-up (in the case of women), are probably the source of the first impression made on a respondent. Since physical appearance can place an interviewer, rightly or wrongly, in some class, such as an economic or opinion class, and since this can have a biasing effect on an interviewer's responses, it is necessary that physical appearance be as neutral as possible. *Neutral* means that the interviewer might be classed in any of a number of groups: he might be rich or poor, well or poorly educated, Republican or Democrat, religious or not, pro- or anti-segregation, from the city or the farm, like or dislike

baseball, and so forth. In a word, the first impression the interviewer makes should leave him "nameless," and the impression should be maintained throughout the interview.

How one goes about becoming unclassifiable is not an easy matter to specify, for every interviewer varies. The following general points can be made, however.

—a. Clothing should be "average"; that is, of the type that is most usually seen in the locality where the interview is conducted. It should be neither too fashionable nor too plain. The same applies to the accessories of women interviewers.

—b. The personal appearance should also be "average." To give rather extreme examples, men with long sideburns may tend to be perceived by other people as liking rock-and-roll music and having lots of chrome on their cars. On the other hand, crew haircuts might suggest a college education. Women who wear absolutely no make-up or nail polish, probably create an impression of coldness, even of masculinity. These impressions, whether right or wrong, are to be avoided. The interviewer may feel that he is being asked to mask his "personality" by suppressing indications of where he belongs in the social matrix. He is being asked to do exactly this, but he should remember that it is part of doing his job well.

—c. Speech should be carefully controlled. This is particularly important at those times when the interviewer's choice of words and phrasing are not controlled by the questionnaire (e.g., during the introduction). The language used should be neither unusual nor overly simple. Technical terms, such as "market analysis" (which might be used in describing the purpose of a survey), should not be used, nor should long, complex sentences. On the other hand, if an interviewer attempts to correct such tendencies in himself he should be very careful not to over-correct and to use language so patently simple as to be potentially insulting. The use of "just plain English" is best as a rule. If this is occasionally not understood, as with foreign-born or illiterate respondents, adjustments can be made.

The choice of language is not all that should be controlled. Intonation, accent peculiarities, and tell-tale expressions should also be controlled. Since this is something that the interviewer is frequently not aware of, it is part of his supervisor's job to point out the peculiarities and to suggest ways of controlling them.

6. *The interviewer must attempt to obtain an interview at the time of his first call, or, if this is not possible, make definite arrangements to obtain the interview at a later time.* This principle is included to cover two fairly common contingencies. The first is when the respondent is actually contacted on the first call but claims that he is too busy to be interviewed at the time. The claim of being busy may be an attempt to "brush off" the interviewer. If this is judged to be the case the interviewer should give his introduction, being sure to state the purpose and importance of the survey, and try to arouse the respondent's interest. If this is unsuccessful he should try to get a *definite* commitment from the respondent on when he will agree to be interviewed. If the respondent is seen to be really busy (e.g., dressed to go out, in the midst of cooking a meal, having company), a date and time for interview should be agreed upon. The interviewer should then show up punctually for the appointment.

The second contingency is when someone answers the call, but the person to be interviewed is unavailable (e.g., sick, at work, out of town). In this case a general introduction to the survey should be given in order to inform and interest the person answering the call. This is necessary because information about where and when the desired respondent can be contacted will be more easily obtained, and because the interest aroused in this person may be passed on to the respondent, thus facilitating the eventual interview. Sometimes the person answering the interviewer's call will offer to be interviewed instead of the desired respondent. In these cases it is important not to offend the person and to explain in a friendly manner why substitution is not possible (See pages 41-42, 46).

When postponing an interview the interviewer should not forget that his own time is valuable. Any decision he makes should therefore be based partly on this factor.

7. *The interviewer's approach must be flexible.* The principles which have been stated are guides rather than hard-and-fast rules. Although most interviews have much in common, each differs from the others in some respect. The interviewer must learn to perceive the differences between interview situations quickly at the very beginning of the introduction and adjust his introductory remarks accordingly. For example, if a female respondent happened to be working in her flower garden at the time of call and was particularly reticent about being interviewed, it might be appropriate to display interest in her garden in order to "break the ice." Or it might be desirable to simplify the introduction for

an apparently illiterate person. Or, again, remarks on the purpose of the survey might be extended somewhat (without giving away too much) if unusual interest was displayed. However, adapting the interview to the needs of the situation *must* be guided by the principles stated earlier.

B. *Choosing the Setting for the Interview*

Once the interviewer has introduced the survey and the respondent has agreed to answer questions, an appropriate setting for the interview must be chosen. This is usually no problem, for the respondent will invite the interviewer into the living room or some quiet room. It happens fairly often, however, that suitable conditions are not immediately provided. It is therefore useful to specify by a few broad principles what constitutes suitable interview settings and to suggest how these may be obtained.

8. *The interview must be conducted in a quiet, comfortable place.* Since most interviews take one-half hour or more to complete, excluding introductory remarks, and require some thought on the respondent's part, quiet and comfort are desirable. To request this of the respondent may also underline the importance of the survey. These conditions are especially beneficial to the interviewer who conducts many interviews every day, day in and day out.

The living room or parlor is usually well suited for interviewing. On occasion, particularly in the evening, this room might be in use by the respondent's family. It is then desirable to suggest that the interview be given in an unoccupied room, such as the dining room, the sun porch, or the kitchen. When the interviewing is being done on farms, it frequently happens that the respondent is doing an essential chore outside the home. The farmer might be working some "bottom" land one-half mile away and find it inconvenient to be interviewed anywhere else. Under these circumstances, despite less than adequate conditions, it would be best to take the interview on the spot; to insist on doing otherwise would probably alienate the respondent. If circumstances are too untoward—e.g., tractor noise, divided attention of the respondent—the interviewer may be wiser to withdraw after making an appointment for a later time.

9. *The respondent must be interviewed alone.* Unless instructions specify the contrary, as might be the case when a wife and her husband are to be interviewed together or when groups are interviewed, no one but the interviewer and respondent should be present during an interview. The presence of even one other person may influence a respondent's

answers and therefore bias them. There is a tendency for many people to modify the "true" answer to a question so that it is in better accord with what the respondent believes are the answers of the other persons present. If the respondent perceives no difference between his answer and those of others there would be no bias, of course; yet there is no way for the interviewer to know what is going on in the respondent's mind as a result of the presence of other people. Hence, no other people should be present. In this connection it is worth noting that the interviewer potentially has the same biasing effects as other persons; however, he has been trained to appear as neutral as possible so that the respondent will find it difficult to estimate what the interviewer's answers to certain questions might be and therefore will have little basis for modifying his answers.

C. *Using the Questionnaire*

After the survey has been introduced and an appropriate setting has been found the interview proper can begin, using the survey questionnaire in accordance with the set of principles set forth in this section. The questionnaire is the basic tool with which information is obtained in order to reduce the researcher's uncertainty about a particular matter. As mentioned previously the questions it contains have been carefully designed and pretested to obtain valid and reliable answers.

10. *The questions must be asked precisely as specified on the questionnaire.* The major reason for using a questionnaire is to insure comparability of answers, no matter who asks or who answers the questions. If answers to a given question were not comparable, they could not be added or averaged or otherwise treated together and would therefore be useless to the researcher. Consider this example of three interviewers asking questions about income: Interviewer A asks, "What was your gross income from salaries or wages last year?"; B asks, "What was your net income last year?"; and C asks, "How much did you earn last year?" Clearly, the income figures given in answer to these questions could not be added and averaged in order to estimate the average income of the respondents in the preceding year. The figures given in response to A's question would be a gross figure; the response to B's question would be a net figure; and the figure given C might be either gross or net. Furthermore, the figure given A would exclude all income other than that from salaries or wages, whereas the figures given B and C would presumably include income from all sources.

Much more subtle differences in questions may also result in lack of comparability. Consider this example based on an actual survey. Two product brands, X and Y, were being compared for consumer preference. One question asked, "Is X better than Y?" whereas a second asked, "Is Y worse than X?" Logically these two forms of the question are equivalent, yet it was found that the answers to each differed.

It sometimes happens that a question, as worded in the questionnaire, does not "feel comfortable" to the interviewer, who then, willy-nilly, rewords it slightly. *Rewording must be avoided.* If the interviewer finds there are such questions he should practice asking them as written until they do feel natural.

11. *The questions must be asked in the order presented on the questionnaire.* When a questionnaire is constructed careful attention is paid to the order in which questions are asked. The sequence which is finally worked out attempts to provide good continuity from question to question, to achieve a more or less conversational flow, to minimize undesirable effects of one question upon another, and to facilitate the interviewer's task. Any departure from the order may therefore have unwanted consequences.

12. *Every question on the questionnaire must be asked.* If a respondent has already answered a question in the course of answering a preceding one, the question should nonetheless be asked as specified on the questionnaire. In so doing it is good practice to precede the question with a remark, such as, "You have already said something about this, but let me ask you. . ." to show that the interviewer has been attentive. The only instance in which it is permissible, even desirable, to omit a question other than a "skip" question (see below) is when the question requires only a simple factual answer which has already been given. Examples are questions about marital status, age, car ownership, veteran status, TV-set ownership, etc.

On some surveys a number of identical or very similar questions are asked about a number of different objects in the same class. For example, a respondent might be asked whether he "liked, disliked, or had no opinion about" each of a dozen different newspaper comic strips. Sometimes a respondent will say, "Oh, I like 'em all" before his opinion of each has been asked. In these cases it is desirable to ask the remainder of the questions if this can be done without unfavorably affecting rapport.

An exception to the rule that every question must be asked occurs when the questionnaire contains contingent, or "skip," questions. These are questions which are asked only when a certain answer was given to a preceding question. Instructions on when to ask or to skip such questions is always printed on the questionnaire at the appropriate place.

13. *When a question is not understood or is misinterpreted it must be repeated, in the same words, not paraphrased.* If a respondent does not understand a question it should be repeated exactly and completely, perhaps posing it more slowly and prefacing it with something like "Well, let me say it more clearly. . ." or "Well, I mean. . . ." In no circumstances should a question be reworded, paraphrased, or "explained." If after one or two repetitions the respondent still fails to comprehend, it is best to record this fact and to proceed with the next question. The same thing applies to misinterpretation unless there is no doubt about the source of misinterpretation, in which case it is permissible to straighten out the difficulty. For example, when it was found in a recent survey that several respondents were misinterpreting the word "foreign" as "farm," it would have been a good idea to define the bothersome term.

A respondent often says, "I don't know," to a question he does not understand or as a means of giving himself time to think. This type of answer, though sometimes genuine, should not be accepted right away at face value, for repetition of the question or a careful probe may bring forth a more valuable answer. However, an answer should not be *forced* out of a respondent.

Instead of saying, "Don't know," respondents may equivocate or give qualified answers by answering, "Yes, if. . .," "Well, it depends. . .," "No, unless. . .," "Probably not, but. . .," and so on. Such responses clearly indicate the necessity of using clarity or hypothetical probes (see below) in order to determine precisely whether the respondent's response is affirmative or negative.

Since questions are carefully pretested it is seldom that they are not understood. If an interviewer should find that a particular question frequently gives trouble, he should report this fact immediately to his supervisor, who, in turn, will report the difficulty to the researchers. Corrections can then be made before the trouble is irreparable.

14. *Questions which respondents hesitate or refuse to answer initially must be handled tactfully in order not to destroy rapport.* Many surveys contain one or more "sensitive" questions—that is, questions which are quite personal or in some way threaten the respondent. Questions about

family relations, sex, education, and income fall in this category, as do questions about a host of social matters, deviate opinions of which, if they exist, are socially unacceptable. When the interviewer comes to a question he believes may be sensitive to a particular respondent, he should *not* give any hint of this. He should instead ask the question in a matter-of-fact manner, as if it were a very natural question for the respondent to answer honestly and straightforwardly. If the respondent then shows signs of hesitation or refuses to answer, the interviewer may remind him of the confidential nature of answers and tell him that all answers are handled as anonymous statistics. Generally excessive pressure should not be applied to obtain answers, for the answers so obtained are probably not worth the resulting loss of rapport. Most surveys, however, contain a certain number of *key* questions to which answers *must* be obtained, even if rapport is threatened, for these questions are central to the objectives of the survey. Rapport, it must be remembered, is a means, not an end.

It is sometimes possible, at the very end of an interview, to return to a question which was skipped because of the respondent's sensitivity to its subject. This can be done under the guise of going over the interview as a whole, clarifying a certain point, and so on. The interviewer may even prepare the ground for this by saying, "Perhaps we can come back to this later, if you want," at the time he skips the sensitive question. When he does this, he must be sure to record his action.

15. *Instructions to the interviewer on the questionnaire must be carefully followed.* At various places on a questionnaire there are instructions to the interviewer. They are usually in different type from the questions, so as not to be missed. The instructions are of different kinds, a few of which follow.

—a. *Instructions on when, how, and for what to probe.* In order to obtain complete, detailed information about certain subjects the interviewer is instructed to "probe." Probing will be discussed at length below.

—b. *Instructions on decisions about what to ask.* Questionnaires often contain "contingent" questions, which are asked or not asked only if certain answers have been given to one or more previous questions. For example, Question 12 would be asked only if the answer to Question 11 was "Yes," whereas Question 13 would be asked only if the answer to Question 11 was "No."

—c. *Instructions on additional things to do in conjunction with certain questions.* Some questions require that the respondent be presented with objects, lists, pictures, and so forth, in connection with answering the questions. For example, a market survey might require that respondents express their opinions of the odor of a new cake of soap, in which case the interviewer would be instructed to hand the soap to respondents as he asked a question about the soap's odor. Or respondents could be given pictures of new automobile designs and be asked to rank the designs in terms of their personal preference.

—d. *Instructions on how to record certain answers.* Answers to certain types of questions must be recorded in special ways—for example, in tables with several rows and columns. In such cases special instructions are printed on the questionnaire. The subject of recording answers will be elaborated on in a later section.

16. *The questionnaire must be used informally and with ease.* Questions are scientific instruments and should therefore be used precisely, but respondents should not be given the impression that they are being measured, tested, or investigated (even though this is really the case). If this impression is given, the respondent is likely to be self-conscious, to be on his guard, and to give biased answers to some questions or to give "don't know" answers. The interviewer should learn to use the questionnaire in an informal, easy-going manner, without appearing to read too closely the questions printed on the questionnaire. This manner can best be achieved by repeated practice interviews and by reading the questionnaire carefully a number of times before going into the field.

17. *Rapport must be maintained throughout the interview.* Despite initially excellent rapport it is possible that it will be threatened for a variety of reasons—for example, by asking a "sensitive" question. When this happens, the interviewer should take time out to strengthen or re-establish rapport. How this is done will vary from case to case, depending on the cause of the trouble, the respondent, and the nature of the survey. No ready-made rules or techniques can be supplied, but it is often effective to take the respondent's mind off the survey for a moment by talking about some unrelated matter of interest to him. If this is done, care should be taken to provide smooth transitions from questioning to irrelevant discussion and back to questioning. When rapport deteriorates it is also effective to remind the respondent that only *his* opinions or answers are important, that there are no right or wrong, good or bad answers, and that responses are confidential.

D. *Using Probes*

Almost all surveys make use of probes. Probes are devices, usually questions, which elicit information in addition to that given in the first response to a general question. There are two broad classes of probes: those which are printed in question form on the questionnaire and those which are spontaneously made by interviewers. The first class of probes, called *questionnaire probes* here, consists of nothing more than questions following up responses to preceding, more general questions. They can usually be identified by the fact that they are lettered (e.g., 11-a, 11-b) and indented. Their use is governed by the principles which have already been outlined.

The second class of probes, which will be called *interviewer probes,* requires much more diligence, insight, and judgment on the interviewer's part, for the probes must be made up on the spot as the interview requires. They are usually used in connection with responses to *open-end* questions —that is, questions which do not provide fixed response alternatives— although they may follow other kinds of questions (e.g., dichotomous and multiple-choice questions). Six types of probes will be discussed here.

—a. *Completion probes* are used to obtain more information on a response which was too general, vague, or incomplete to be useful. They are attempts to have a respondent *expand* or *give more details* on his original response. Examples of completion probes are: "Anything else?" "Could you tell me more about that?" "What else can you think of?" "Does anything else come to your mind?"

—b. *Clarity probes* are also used to elicit additional information on a preceding response, but in contrast to completion probes they press the respondent to *explain* a response which was unclear, lacked a referent, or did not make sense in the context of the question. Typical clarity probes are: "I don't quite see what you mean," "Could you explain that a little more?" "Could you give me an example of that?" "Why is that?" Some probes may, of course, be more specific and partially repeat something the respondent said. For example, when a female respondent was asked, "Why is it that you shop at the Speedway Store rather than at some other store?" she answered, "It's more convenient to shop there." Unfortunately, "convenient" may mean many things: the store may have a comprehensive selection of merchandise, or it may allow charge accounts, or it may be close to home. Therefore, to clarify the response, a probe such as "Could you explain what you mean by 'convenient?'" would have been appropriate.

—c. *Channel probes* are used to uncover or trace back the source of an opinion or to define a vague referent. They serve to distinguish between an original and an adopted opinion, as well as to specify the source of a reported opinion. In response to the question, "A lot of people are talking about taxes these days. Do you think they are going up, down, or are going to stay the same?" a respondent might say, for example, "I've heard that the State is going to increase income taxes next year." An appropriate channel probe could be, "Where have you heard that?" Or, a respondent might say, "I think taxes are going up. They say it's bound to happen." In this case it would be important to probe and find out who are "they" by asking, "whom do you mean by 'they?'" Sometimes it is not immediately possible to use a channel probe because the response does not provide a ready-made basis for it (as "they" in the last example). It is therefore necessary to use another type of probe first. For the sake of illustration, let us assume a respondent answered to the above question, "I think taxes are going up." The interviewer might then ask, "Why do you think that?" (clarity probe) to which the respondent might answer, "Oh, that's what people say hereabouts." The latter answer would be an ideal set-up for a channel probe—for instance, "What people do you mean?"

—d. *Hypothetical probes* are very fruitful devices but must be made up and used with great care. They consist in presenting hypothetical situations or events and having the respondent react to them. As with other types of probes, they must be based on the respondent's previous answer —that is to say, *the hypothetical situation or event must have been suggested or implied by the respondent himself.* For example, in a recent survey individuals were asked, "Do you think Red China should be given a seat in the United Nations or not?" One respondent answered, "I don't think Red China should be given a seat in the U.N. as long as they have anything to do with Russia." An appropriate hypothetical probe in this instance would have been, "Well, what if they broke with Russia?" In general, hypothetical probes can be used whenever a response implies an alternative condition or state of affairs.

—e. *Reactive probes* are employed primarily to elicit affective reactions or feelings to situations which have been mentioned by the respondent. For instance, in a survey about child rearing a respondent might have said, "We firmly believe children should be punished," to the question, "How do you feel about disciplining children?" A probe such as, "How do you personally feel about punishing children?" might then have resulted in the respondent's replying, "I hate it, myself." Thus the probe would have brought out important additional information.

—f. *High-pressure probes* must be used *cautiously* and *only* when rapport is very strong. They serve to pin down a respondent who is suspected of having given a purely platitudinous answer to a question or to resolve contradictions in the interview. In a study of anti-Semitism, for example, a respondent might have said, "All people have equal rights," to the question, "Do you think it is fair or unfair not to hire people solely because they are Jewish?" Because of other responses the interviewer might suspect that this was no more than lip service to an ideal. If rapport was good, he might then ask, "Is that what you *really* think?" or, "Do *you*, personally, think that applies to Jewish people?" As a rule the high-pressure probe should be strictly limited to cases where nothing else will elicit the desired information *and* where rapport is strong.

The six types of interviewer probes which have been discussed are necessary tools of interviewers, and their use should be practiced before every survey. Because of the great variety of contingencies in which they can be used, it is impossible to specify exactly what probes should be used at what point in an interview. If this were possible, the probes would be printed on the questionnaire. It is possible, however, to state certain broad principles governing their use.

18. *Probes must be used* (a) *when the response is irrelevant to the question asked,* (b) *when an answer is unclear,* (c) *when an answer seems incomplete, and* (d) *when an answer is suspected of being untrue.* This principle needs no elaboration beyond stating that before it can apply the interviewer must know the objectives of questions and learn to recognize unclear, incomplete, and fallacious answers when they occur.

19. *Probes must not suggest responses.* An interviewer often knows (or thinks he knows) what a respondent means, how he feels, and what his real opinion is, even though the respondent has not expressed these things. He is therefore tempted to suggest them in his probing. This must be avoided absolutely, for an interviewer's suggestion may be accepted by the respondent and be recorded as the latter's own thought, when, in fact, it is the interviewer's. There is no way of knowing what a respondent means, feels, or thinks until he, himself, expresses it. As has already been noted, the suggestion of answers can be avoided by using completely nondirective probes (e.g., "Anything else?") or by basing a probe on the content of the respondent's previous answer (e.g., "How do you personally feel about punishing children?").

20. *The use of probes presumes good rapport and requires tact.* Probes by nature tend to press or challenge a respondent and therefore potentially may unfavorably affect an interview. Hence, it is necessary that good rapport exist before probes are put to use and, when they are used, that probing be tactful.

E. *Closing the Interview*

After the questioning phase of the interview has been completed the questionnaire should be briefly reviewed in the presence of the respondent to make certain that all required information has been obtained and recorded. If some questions were deliberately skipped because they threatened rapport, an attempt to obtain answers to them should be made during the review. Similarly, inconsistencies between responses may be resolved. It should be noted, however, that inconsistencies may actually represent the way a respondent thinks. Care must therefore be taken not to *force* consistency.

21. *The respondent must be thanked for his participation in the survey and be left with a feeling that the interview has been a pleasant and interesting experience.* This is important, for even though a given respondent may never again be interviewed, his attitude toward surveys contributes to that of the general public. In a sense, then, the interviewer partly determines the reception he will get on subsequent interviews. In cases where the survey design calls for one or more re-interviews, as in panel studies, respondents not only should be thanked for their cooperation in the interview just completed but should also be prepared for later interviews (unless there are instructions to the contrary) by being told that additional information would be appreciated and that the interviewer will return another day.

F. *Recording Responses*

The interviewer is the researcher's agent and serves as an intermediary between him and the respondent. He communicates the researcher's needs (via questions) to the respondent and then communicates the information obtained back to the researcher. For the latter communication to be effective it is necessary that the responses obtained be appropriately recorded on the questionnaire. The ideal goal towards which to strive is having the recorded responses as meaningful to the researcher as if he had done the interviewing himself. Following a few general principles will help to achieve this ideal.

22. Responses must be recorded at the time they are made. Practice has shown conclusively that responses which are recorded *after* the interview are distorted, if not totally in error. They should therefore be recorded as completely as possible on the spot.

23. A respondent's own words must be recorded. In order that responses be as meaningful as possible to the researcher they must be recorded *verbatim*. Since answers to most questions are fairly brief, this can easily be done. However, some answers to open-end questions are quite long and spoken rapidly, making it difficult for the interviewer to attend to the response and to record it simultaneously. In such cases the *substance* and *meaning* of a response must be accurately recorded. Abbreviations should be avoided. Whenever it is essential to have verbatim records the researcher will provide the interviewer with a recording aid, such as a tape recorder, and give him appropriate training in how to use it effectively.

24. Non-responses must be accounted for in detail. A question which a respondent could not or would not answer should not be left blank. The reason for not responding should be given in as much detail as possible. If a respondent did not understand a question, for example, the interviewer should specify what it was he did not understand. In cases of refusal, the reason for refusing to answer should be specified, if it can be determined. When reasons for non-responses are recorded the researcher is able to learn something about the respondent, as well as about the instruments he designed.

25. All interviewer probes must be recorded in parentheses. Responses are meaningful only when the stimuli which elicited them are known. Thus the response, "I hate it, myself," is totally meaningless unless it is known that it followed the probe, "How do you personally feel about punishing children?" Response-probe-response sequences should be fully recorded in the proper order, with the probes in parentheses. Parentheses should be used for no other purpose than to identify probes.

26. Significant events during the course of the interview must be recorded. Significant events are those which have had or may have an effect on the interview. Major interruptions, emotional reactions, changes in rapport, lapses of attention, and special signs of interest are examples of significant events. Since they may help in interpreting an interview they should be reported at the point where they occur in the interview.

27. *Recorded responses must be clearly legible.*

28. *Before a questionnaire is returned to the supervisor it must be checked for completeness, understandability, and legibility.*

CHAPTER IV

Sampling

In its most general sense, sampling refers to selecting from a universe of units a portion of the units which, as a group, is representative of the entire universe. The purpose of sampling is to estimate economically and accurately characteristics of a universe by measuring those characteristics on a sample of units. In presidential pre-election polls a sample of 2,500-5,000 adult persons is selected from the universe of adult persons in the United States, and the voting intentions of the persons in the sample are used to estimate the voting intentions of the universe. In cotton-growing states a sample of cotton farms is selected from the universe of cotton farms to estimate the size and quality of the cotton crop before harvest. Television program preferences are estimated from the preferences of a sample of TV-set owners selected from the universe of TV-set owners.

If a sample is to be representative of the universe from which it is drawn, the sampling procedures must prevent the intrusion of the subjective (often unconscious) preferences of a human agent, such as those of an interviewer. In practice selection is often done by use of random numbers in conjunction with a rigid procedure which does not allow subjectivity to intrude.

The role of the interviewer in the sampling phase varies with the type of sample and the specifications of the universe being sampled. In some surveys the interviewer does not participate in the sampling phase. The respondent may be designated by name from a list of all possible respondents, or the exact address of a household might be furnished for the subsequent identification of the respondent. The use of *area probability* sampling methods, however, often requires the interviewer to make the final identification of the sampling units and respondents as a part of the field work.

The following example of area probability sampling and procedures is given as one of a number of possible procedures which might be used in the field identification of sampling units and respondents.

A. *Introduction to Area Probability Sampling*

With the area probability method, sampling of the unit of observation (usually an individual) is accomplished in several stages, some of which are carried out in the research office and others of which are carried out by the interviewer in the field.*

For the sake of illustration, let it be assumed that the sampling problem is to select a sample of adult persons, 18 years of age or more, from the state of North Carolina. We begin with the (verifiable) assumption that every adult can be associated with one, and only one, *occupied dwelling unit* (ODU) which, in turn, can be associated with one, and only one, *area segment* of land. When an adult is associated with several ODU's uniform rules are made which will result in his being associated with only one of these. Similarly, rules are made to take care of ODU's which are associated with more than one area segment, as when a dwelling unit straddles two segments.

The general procedures for selecting an area probability sample are illustrated by the following example:

1. The state of North Carolina is divided into 100 politico-geographic county units, which are mutually exclusive. A sample of these *counties* is drawn according to the sample design.

2. Each selected county is then arbitrarily divided (in the office) into mutually exclusive area segments consisting of blocks (in cities and towns) and land areas bounded by roads, railroad tracks, streams, and so forth (in the open country outside of cities and towns). A sample of these *area segments* is then selected from each county by a specified procedure.

3. Each area segment contains within its boundaries a number of occupied dwelling units (ODU's). A sample of these ODU's is selected from each segment by a prescribed procedure.

4. In each ODU† there reside one or more adults. A sample of one or more *adults* in each ODU is selected according to rule.

---

* Strictly speaking, all *selection* of the sample is conducted in the research office because occupied dwelling units (ODU's) and individuals in the sample are specified by instructing the interviewer. For example, the interviewer is instructed to contact ODU #2 and to interview adult #3 in that ODU. It is then the job of the interviewer to *locate* that ODU and individual in the field. The researcher, of course, does not know the address of ODU #2 nor the name of adult #3, but if his instructions are followed exactly the same ODU and adult will always be located no matter who the interviewer is.

† One ODU is occupied by one *household*. One household is the collection of persons living in one ODU. See Glossary for complete definitions.

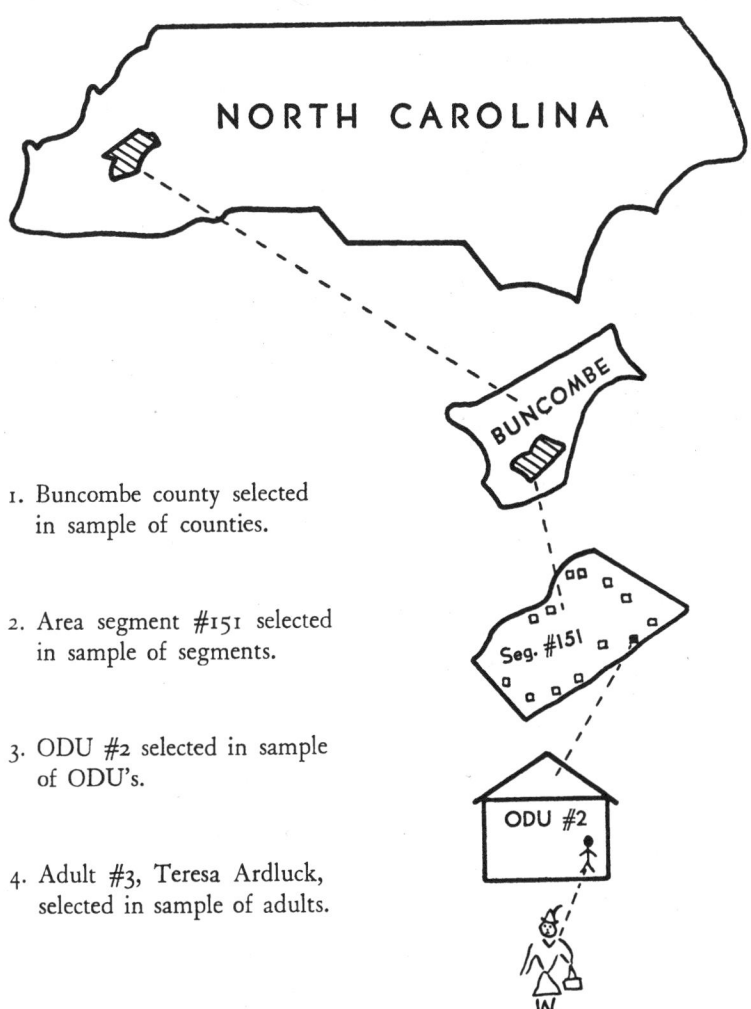

NORTH CAROLINA

1. Buncombe county selected in sample of counties.

2. Area segment #151 selected in sample of segments.

3. ODU #2 selected in sample of ODU's.

4. Adult #3, Teresa Ardluck, selected in sample of adults.

FIGURE 1. EXAMPLE OF SAMPLING IN FOUR STAGES

The four-step procedure described above is illustrated in Figure 1, which shows how one county is selected from the state, one segment from the county, one ODU from the segment, and one adult from the ODU.

In actual practice more than one county, segment, household, and adult would be selected. The first two steps of sampling are accomplished in the research office. As a result, the interviewer is given the selected area segments in which he must carry out the third and fourth steps of sampling. The remainder of this chapter will describe in detail the selection procedures to be used by interviewers. *These procedures must be followed to the letter if selected samples are to have a chance of being representative.*

B. *Identifying the Sample ODU's*

Each interviewer is given maps, or aerial photos, or both, on which the area segments assigned to him are delineated and numbered. In addition he is given Segment Sketch Sheets, ODU Identification Sheets, and Individual Identification Sheets. For each area segment assigned to him the interviewer should proceed as follows:

1. The segment should be located beyond doubt by going around it. This is usually easily done since segments are bounded by identifiable landmarks such as streets, roads, railroad tracks, streams, rivers, or power lines, whenever possible. In the open country, bridges, churches, schools, and road map distances are also used. Map reading will be facilitated by carefully studying the standard symbols printed on maps.

2. A large sketch of the segment should be made. The sketch should be properly oriented with respect to the North arrow on the Segment Sketch Sheet (SSS) and should show the major landmarks bounding the segment. The interviewer should go to the northeast corner of the segment (or the easternmost of the northern points if the northeast corner is difficult to identify) and, while "cruising," mark with a cross (X) the location of all ODU's *inside* the segment on the SSS. Similarly, the location of vacant dwellings should be marked with O's. Since some structures (e.g., a house) may contain more than one dwelling unit, it is important that such things as separate entrances, number of mail boxes, and number of TV antennas be noticed. A plurality of these usually indicates more than one dwelling within the structure. Whenever a structure contains more than one dwelling unit, as many X's should be marked on the sketch as there are dwellings. If streets, roads, alleys, or paths run *into or through* the segment, they should be explored and drawn on the SSS (in the country, a dirt road may lead to a farmhouse not visible from the main road).

3. Having indicated on the SSS the location of all dwelling units, the interviewer should then number all ODU's consecutively in a clockwise direction, starting with the one nearest the northeast corner of the segment. If there are two or more dwellings in a single structure the lowest numbered addresses or apartment should be numbered first, then the others should be numbered in ascending order of address or apartment

number. If the addresses are the same and the dwelling units are not numbered, numbering should proceed from the bottom floor to the top floor, starting on the left of the first floor (the basement is considered the first floor) and proceeding around in a clockwise, upward spiral direction. An example of a completed SSS is shown in Figure 2.

INTERVIEWER: Matilda Trotz   SEGMENT No. 151-2-3

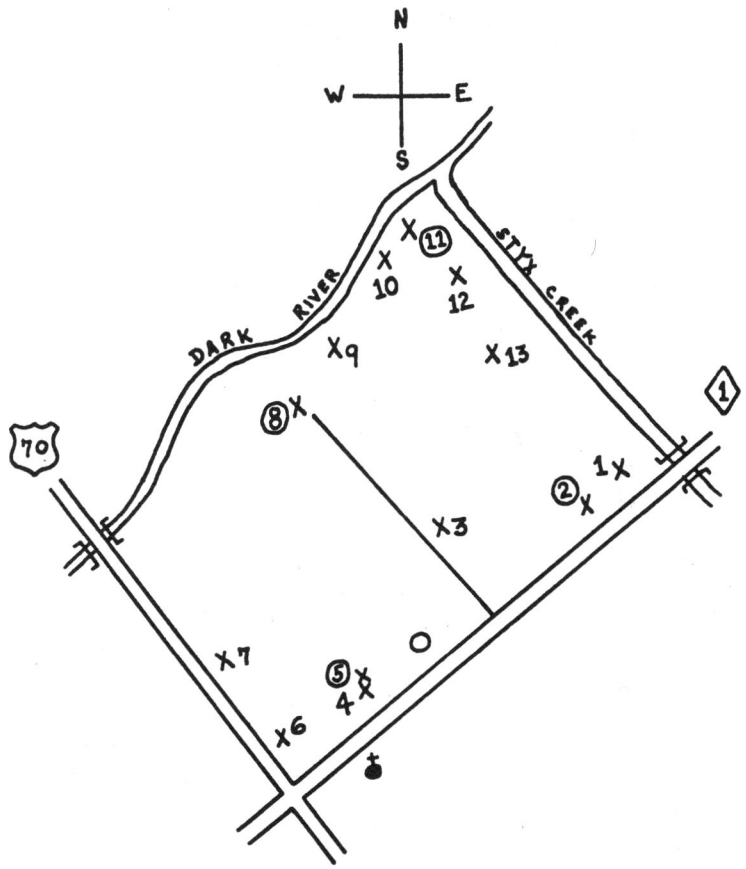

FIGURE 2. EXAMPLE OF A COMPLETED SEGMENT SKETCH SHEET

4. The next step is to determine which ODU's in the segment are designated for the sample. The second and third numbers of the three numbers identifying the segment on the interviewer's map or photo determine this, while the first identifies the segment proper. The number on the map or photo might be 151-2-3, for example. The second number,

2, designates ODU #2 as the first ODU in the sample. This number should be circled on the SSS (See Figure 2). The third number in 151-2-3 is 3 and indicates that every *third* ODU after ODU #2 is also in the sample. The number of each ODU so selected should be circled on the SSS. In the example in Figure 2, ODU's #2, #5, #8, and #11 are in the sample and circled on the SSS.

5. After the sample ODU's have been identified on the SSS, the ODU Identification Sheet (IDS) should be filled out (this may be done at the same time that the SSS is completed, if the interviewer is reasonably

ODU IDENTIFICATION SHEET

INTERVIEWER Matilda Trotz   SEGMENT No. 151

ODU #'S IN SAMPLE 2, 5, 8, etc.

ODU No.	Name of Head of Household	Action*	ODU No.	Name of Head of Household	Action*
1	Paul Retch		16		
②	John Ardluck	C	17		
3	D. C. Washington		18		
4	Irving Hope		19		
⑤	Desper Attmeany	NC	20		
6	Mrs. Flora Jolly	SC	21		
7	Alfred Rex		22		
⑧	Smiley Katz	C	23		
9	Lance Lotte		24		
10	Joe Gazzo		25		
⑪	Hardie Sonn	C	26		
12	Alan George		27		
13	Branch Waters		28		
14			29		
15			30		

*C—contacted; NC—not contacted; SC—substitute contact.

FIGURE 3. Example of Completed ODU Identification Sheet

certain that no dwelling units have been missed). The IDS serves to identify by name every ODU in the segment and to indicate what action was taken with each. As on the SSS, the numbers of the ODU's in the sample should be circled. In many cases the name of the head of household in each ODU can be ascertained from mail boxes or name plates without actually knocking at every door. Of course a call is eventually made at every *sample* ODU, and it is then possible to complete missing information by asking the names of neighbors. In Figure 3, for example, if the name of the head of household in ODU #3 could not be ascertained initially, the information could probably be obtained when calling at sample ODU #2.

The above procedure is basic to sampling ODU's and can be followed exactly if all ODU's in a segment have been correctly identified when "cruising." However, it sometimes happens that all ODU's are not identified or that some vacant dwellings have been marked as occupied. When this occurs it is necessary to modify the procedure somewhat. Segment 151-2-3 may be taken as an example. Let it be assumed that the interviewer has called at ODU #2 and that he has asked whether ODU's #1, #3, and #4 are really single dwelling units or whether they are multiple dwelling units. He finds out that ODU's #1 and #4 are single ODU's but that ODU #3 is actually a two-dwelling-unit duplex. This requires that the SSS and IDS be renumbered, that a new ODU be added, and that a new sample of ODU's be identified (except for ODU's #1 and #2, which retain their original numbers).

The procedure for selecting ODU's may be summarized by the following steps:

a. *The segment must be located and "cruised."*

b. *A sketch of the segment, showing the boundaries and major landmarks, must be made on the Segment Sketch Sheet (SSS).*

c. *Beginning at the northeast corner of the segment, all ODU's must be marked and numbered in clockwise, consecutive order on the SSS.*

d. *The numbers of the ODU's designated in the sample must be identified and circled on the SSS.*

e. *The ODU Identification Sheet must be filled out, listing all ODU's and the names of heads of households, and showing which are in the sample.*

C. *Selecting Individuals*

In some surveys only one unspecified individual, or the head of the household, or the housewife is to be interviewed, and there is, therefore, no sampling to be done within an ODU. Frequently a sample of individuals from a designated universe (e.g., individuals 18 years of age or more living in sample ODU's) is to be identified *after* the sample of ODU's has been designated. The procedure for doing this will be described in this section, using as an example the universe of individuals 18 years of age or more living in ODU #2, Segment 151-2-3. The example can, of course, be generalized to other universes, such as adult females, children, unmarried males, or household domestics.

1. The interviewer calls at ODU #2, makes his introductory remarks to Teresa Ardluck, who opens the door, and asks her who the head of

INDIVIDUAL IDENTIFICATION SHEET

INTERVIEWER Matilda Trotz   SEGMENT No. 151

ODU No.   2

INDIVIDUALS IN SAMPLE 1, 3, 5, etc.

Ind. No.	Age	Name	Relationship to Head	Action*
4	31	John Ardluck	Head	
③	33	Teresa Ardluck	Wife	I
①	56	Abigail Adams	Mother-in-law	NI
⑤	29	Sissy Adams	Sister-in-law	I
	8	Paul Ardluck	Son	
2	47	Aston Ragtail	Roomer	SI
	5	Peggy Ardluck	Daughter	
6	26	Peter Adams	Brother-in-law	
⑦	24	Juniper Adams	Sister-in-law	I

*I—interviewed, NI—not interviewed, SI—substitute interview.

FIGURE 4. Example of Completed Individual Identification Sheet

household is and who the other occupants are. He records the names of the occupants on the Individual Identification Sheet (INID), beginning with the head of household. He then asks the age of each occupant and the relationship of each to the head, and records the obtained information in the appropriate columns on the INID (see Figure 4).

2. The interviewer numbers all persons 18 years of age or more by age rank. In the example of Figure 4, Abigail Adams is #1 since she is the oldest, Aston Ragtail is #2 since he is second oldest, and so on. The two children are not numbered, since in this example they are outside the universe of persons 18 years old or older.

3. The interviewer next looks at the top of the INID to find out which individuals are in the sample—in this example individuals #1, #3, #5, and #7, or every odd-numbered one. These numbers are circled in the first column and interviewing may again begin with Teresa Ardluck, since she is in the sample and the interviewer is already talking with her.

The procedure just described is straightforward and closely parallels the procedure for sampling ODU's. The procedure can be summarized as follows:

a. *The names, ages, and relationships to head of household of all persons living in a sample ODU must be recorded on the Individual Identification Sheet* (INID).

b. *The individuals in the universe to be sampled must be numbered by age rank.*

c. *The numbers of the individuals to be in the sample must be determined from the top of the INID and circled.*

D. *Special Rules*

The preceding procedures for selecting sample ODU's and individuals, though basic and sufficient to handle most instances, make no provisions for cases where an ODU or an individual cannot be contacted. Such cases might call for special rules, of which the following are only examples. Two rules are described here: one to cover instances in which no *initial contact* can be made with a sample ODU or individual (Callback Rule), and one to cover instances in which *no contact at all* can be made with a sample ODU or individual (Substitution Rule).

1. *Call-back Rule: If sample ODU's or individuals cannot be contacted on the first call and there is no information indicating that they cannot be contacted, two additional calls must be made before invoking the Substitution Rule.* It occasionally happens that all occupants of a sample ODU are away, or that an individual designated for interview is

unavailable. When this occurs the interviewer should try to obtain information (e.g., from neighbors) about the ODU or individual to determine whether contact can be made within a reasonable period of time, and if it is thought that contact can be made, when it can be made. If it is believed contact can be made—or, more precisely, if there is no reason pointing to the contrary—two more attempts should be made to establish contact. If, on the other hand, there is trustworthy information indicating that no contact can be made within a reasonable period of time (e.g., family away on vacation, individual is sick), the Substitution Rule can be invoked unless instructed otherwise. Resort can also be made to this rule after the third unsuccessful contact.

When the interviewer makes call-backs he should time them to maximize the likelihood of establishing contact. If the problem is that of not being able to contact an ODU because no one is home, information on the best time to call back can usually be obtained from neighbors. When such information is unavailable, calling back one-half to one hour after local working hours will often result in contact. If the distance to the ODU is great, the telephone may be used for establishing contact. If the problem is that of contacting an individual from an ODU with which contact has been made, reliable information on when to call again can usually be obtained from other occupants.

2. *Substitution Rule: If it has been resolved that an ODU cannot be contacted or that an individual cannot be interviewed, the next higher numbered ODU or individual can be substituted unless instructed otherwise.* Information that an ODU or individual cannot be contacted might be obtained from neighbors or other occupants of the ODU. Three unsuccessful calls at the ODU or on the individual would also establish unavailability. The *next higher numbered* ODU or individual refers to the numbering on the IDS and the INID. The columns labeled "Action" in Figures 3 and 4 give examples of substitution. In Figure 3 the ODU of Desper Attmeany could not be "contacted" because of a death in the family (Action: NC). The next higher numbered ODU, the home of Mrs. Flora Jolly, was therefore contacted (Action: SC). In Figure 4 it was found that Abigail Adams was visiting a distant relative in New England and would not be back for several weeks (Action: NI). The roomer, Aston Ragtail, was interviewed instead since he was the next higher numbered individual (Action: SI).

Occasionally there is no "next higher numbered" ODU or individual to substitute (e.g., Juniper Adams is the highest numbered individual in Figure 4). In such cases the next lower numbered ODU or individual must be substituted (e.g., Peter Adams, if Juniper was unavailable).

A modification in the Substitution Rule is made when an upper limit is placed upon the number of interviews to be obtained in any one segment, and the number of ODU's in the segment designated for the sample exceeds the limit. In such a case the next higher numbered *designated* sample ODU is substituted rather than the next higher numbered ODU. The following hypothetical instance will illustrate the procedure: the segment number on the interviewer's map is 386-1-2, meaning that in segment 386 every second ODU, beginning with ODU #1, is to be selected for the sample. The interviewer locates the segment, sketches it, and marks 17 ODU's. He correctly circles ODU's #1, #3, #5, #7, #9, #11, #13, #15, and #17 on the SSS and IDS as those falling in the sample. However, because an arbitrary limit of six interviews per segment had been established, only ODU's #1, #3, #5, #7, #9, and #11 need be contacted. The interviewer contacts and obtains interviews in ODU's #1, #3, #5, #7, and #11, but after three unsuccessful calls at ODU #9 he has to substitute. The ODU to be substituted is #13, the ODU which would have normally fallen in the sample had there not been a limit of six interviews per segment.

There are instances where no substitutions are allowed. In these cases the Call-back Rule is in effect—or a similar rule is—and no substitution is effected. The interviewer will always be given specific instructions in regard to substitution.

CHAPTER V

Common Sources of Interviewer Bias

A variety of sources of interviewer biases have been pointed out in preceding chapters. Discussion of them was kept to a minimum while emphasis was put upon principles of interviewing and sampling. In this chapter the major known sources of interviewer biases will be discussed in greater detail with the hope that the interviewer who becomes aware of common biases will be in a better position to control them. It must be pointed out that by no means are all sources of bias known, for many sources are so subtle as to have escaped observation. Thus, the sources presented here are the more obvious, grosser ones and, by the same token, probably the most important ones.

Bias results from a constant, systematic type of error and is distinguished from a variable, random type of error. Variable errors are those which, on the average and over a large number of measurements, add to zero. This is because, on the average, some of the errors of measurement will be somewhat above the true measurement, whereas others will be somewhat lower. Constant errors, on the other hand, result from consistently making measurements which are above or which are below the true measurement. The following illustration will make clear the distinction between the two types of errors. Let it be supposed that Matilda Trotz, whose "true" weight was exactly 140 pounds all the time, weighed herself three times each day for three days on the bathroom scales. The scale readings she made were 139.7, 139.5, 140.2, 140.8, 139.8, 140.1, 138.9, 140.5, and 140.5 pounds. Every one of these weight measurements is in error since none is exactly 140 pounds, but the *average* of the weights is 140 pounds. Thus the errors are variable errors and the average of the nine measurements is an unbiased estimate of the interviewer's weight. But let it be supposed now that Matilda's weight was exactly 141 pounds and that the measurements she made were the same as before. The measurement errors now not only vary from weighing to weighing but are constant errors as well, because, on the average, they underestimate Matilda's weight by one pound. They are biased measurements. If Matilda investigated a little she might find the scale pointer registered minus one pound instead of zero when the scale was unloaded. This error in the scale would be the source of bias—that is, the cause of constant errors. The source of bias could have been, of course, Matilda Trotz herself. If she were a weight-conscious female she might have consistently misread the scale by one pound. In interviewing, the sources of bias are not so readily isolated. They exist, nevertheless, and the most important ones will now be discussed in the approximate order in which they are likely to occur.

A. *Failure to List Completely*

It has been found by the Bureau of the Census, as well as by a number of private organizations and institutions using area probability samples, that the results of many surveys are biased because interviewers fail to list completely either ODU's or, in fewer cases, individuals within ODU's. The bias results not so much from the fact that, by not being listed, all ODU's did not have an equal chance of being selected for the sample, but from the fact that those not listed tend to be somewhat different from those listed. For example, ODU's which are not listed are likely to be garage and basement apartments, dwellings in multiple-dwelling houses, dwellings far back from the street or road, and so forth. Associated with such dwellings are people whose income might be lower than the neighborhood average, or who are perhaps younger than average and childless. If such people are not given a chance to enter the sample, estimates of income, age, and family size based on the obtained sample will be greater than they should be. They will be biased estimates.

The same type of bias would result from failing to list individuals living in an ODU. For example, sometimes new-born and very young children in large families are not listed, because apparently they are so "new" that they are momentarily forgotten by the parents. It is obvious that if the survey sample includes children, bias will result when the interviewer omits some children on his INID. Other individuals who may not be listed are those who are psychologically not part of the family, though they are members of the household. Roomers, people who travel frequently, recluses, and domestics are examples.

The failure to list all ODU's in a segment usually results from (1) the failure to investigate a segment thoroughly at the time the segment sketch is made, and (2) the failure to ask appropriate questions about neighboring dwellings from persons in the segment. The first failure can be corrected by going into all alleys, dirt roads, side streets, and drives which are within the segment when the segment is being cruised. Structures about which the interviewer is in doubt should be investigated by making inquiries. Similarly, inquiries should be made about all dwellings which may contain more than one dwelling unit—for example, large houses, places with more than one mail box, television antenna, or entrance, and dwellings with fractional street numbers. After this investigation has been made and the interviewer begins to contact sample ODU's, inquiries should be made about dwellings on either side of the one contacted. In the example given previously on page 36, if the interviewer were to contact ODU's #2, #5, #8, and #11, he would ask the person contacted in ODU #2 whether #1, #3, and #4 were single ODU's. When contacting #5 he would obtain similar information about #6 and #7, and so on. With this procedure the probability of missing an ODU would be very small, if not reduced to zero.

Although the failure to list individuals living in an ODU occurs less frequently than the failure to list ODU's, precautions must nevertheless be taken. The best safeguard is to probe thoroughly when obtaining information about household members: "Is there any one else living here?" "Are there any other children besides those you named?" "Any servants living in the house?" It should be noted that probing in this instance may be directive—that is, the probes may suggest persons who might have been omitted from the list, such as servants, roomers, and children.

B. *Failure to Get Designated ODU's and Individuals*

As has been previously mentioned, substitution is permissible only as a last resort, after every reasonable effort has been made to contact an ODU or to interview an individual. The reason that substitution must be strictly limited is that ODU's and individuals for which substitutions are made may have different characteristics than the substitutes. In one recent North Carolina market area survey, for example, it was found that the ODU's most difficult to contact were inhabited by childless families, both members of which worked during the day and whose shopping habits were quite different from those of other families in the sample. If substitutions had been made for many of these families, the estimates of the shopping habits of the universe studied would have been seriously biased. In general, if there is a correlation between the ability to contact ODU's or to interview individuals and a characteristic being studied (e.g., shopping habits), biased estimates will result from substitution. The degree of bias will vary with the number of substitutions made.

Except where substitution is not permitted, legitimate reasons for substituting ODU's are absence of all occupants for a period too long to permit a call-back, serious and contagious illnesses, death in the family, refusal to participate in the survey, and unavailability after a certain number of calls. The same reasons apply to substituting individuals, with the additional reason (unless otherwise specified) that individuals may usually be substituted if they cannot adequately communicate with the interviewer—that is, if they are insane, deaf and dumb, or unable to understand and speak English. This does not, of course, apply to children, with whom communication is often difficult. Special training is usually required and given when young children are to be interviewed. Of the several reasons for substitution, refusals and unavailability after three calls are relatively major problems. They are problems because many interviewers accept refusals too easily, and because in their eagerness to get on with the job they do not time call-backs properly.

It is a commonly observed fact that some interviewers report many more refusals than do others, and the disproportion cannot entirely be accounted for by differences in assignments. What probably does account for differences in refusals is that interviewers with high refusal rates make inadequate introductions, and when refusals are encountered they accept them too easily. *The introduction must be perfected,* for this will not only reduce refusals, but will also make it easier to change a person's mind *after* he has initially refused to cooperate. In perfecting the introduction special care should be taken:

1. Not to create an impression that the interviewer is a salesman.

2. Not to threaten a person with the possibility of being investigated or tested. Indeed, the words "investigated" and "tested" should not be used for that reason. Suggestions that a survey is a psychological study or a study of intelligence or knowledge should also be avoided.

3. To arouse interest in the subject of the survey, by emphasizing those parts which are likely to be of most interest to the person. In consumer surveys, for example, there are usually enough different products covered to interest anyone. With a male person automobiles could be stressed, while with an elderly woman food products could be emphasized. This should not be overdone, however, to the point that the context of the survey is vastly different with different respondents.

4. To establish the impression that the person would be participating

in something important and would be making a contribution if he cooperated with the interviewer.

Although interviewers are usually commendably in a hurry to complete contacts and interviews in an area segment and to move on to the next, their desire for completion frequently results in substitution when none would have been necessary had they timed their call-backs so as to maximize success. Choosing the optimal times for call-back requires prior information about the ODU or individual, though the most general sort of information may be sufficient. Housewives who are away during the morning or afternoon usually return home to prepare noon or evening meals. Men who work away from home during the day can usually be located at home after six. If they are likely to be commuters, somewhat more time must be allowed for their return home. When calling on these individuals, however, great care should be taken to prevent annoyance, for often a housewife returning from a shopping trip or a man coming from work will be tired and not wish to be bothered. In such cases the interviewer's introductory remarks might include a word of apology and offer to arrange a time for interview which is convenient to the prospective respondent. As mentioned previously, appointments can be made by telephone when it is definitely more economical to do so, but it should be noted that personal contact is always more effective and therefore to be preferred. Unless the survey specifies that interviews take place in the home, as might be necessary in consumer studies which include kitchen cupboard checks, the interviewer may find it convenient and economical to interview an individual at his place of work. Before doing so, however, the individual's permission must be asked (e.g., by telephone) in order not to embarrass him should visitors not be allowed during business hours.

The rule which specifies that two call-backs in addition to the initial call must be made before substituting, unless there is unequivocal evidence that contact or an interview is not possible, is to insure that sample specifications will be met. If call-backs are not appropriately timed the rule loses its purpose. Timing should be calculated and not be just a chance affair.

C. Suggesting Responses

An undoubtedly common, but difficult to assess, source of bias is the suggesting of responses by the interviewer. The suggestions may be direct or indirect. Direct suggestions are those which are actually verbalized, whereas indirect ones result from the attitudes, demeanor, and characteristics of the interviewer. The two types will be discussed separately.

The direct suggestion of responses is most likely to occur during probing, when the interviewer is not using carefully designed questions. Direct suggestions may suggest very specific responses or may suggest a general dimension of response. For instance, while probing for the reason that the respondent intends to support the Republican ticket, the interviewer might say "Is that because of the graft in Washington?" thus suggesting a very specific reason. On the other hand, while in a similar situation, the interviewer might probe with the question, "Is that because of the way you feel about the Democratic Administration?" This probe, in contrast to the specificity of former, suggests a negative affective response which could take on a variety of specific aspects. Any probe which suggests either a response or an avenue of response is to be avoided, unless, of course, the response was implied by the respondent himself.

The indirect suggestion of response is a very subtle affair and is difficult to specify in any one case. Nevertheless it does occur, and the resulting bias may be very serious when all interviews in a survey are considered together. The effect of indirect suggestion results from the fact that respondents frequently adjust their "true" responses, especially on questions of opinion, in accordance with the perceived demands of the situation. Generally, if there is a discrepancy between what respondents personally think and what they believe the interviewer thinks, they will give a response which minimizes the discrepancy. A few individuals will do just the opposite; that is, they will exaggerate the discrepancy or make one. Because of this tendency it is desirable that respondents be given no clue of what the interviewer might think. Furthermore, the clue need not be as obvious as an "I Like Ike" button, a Phi Beta Kappa key, or a Masonic Lodge ring. *Apparent* education, social status, income, or ethnic origin are used as clues to a variety of opinions. Opinions about one subject serve as clues to other opinions. For example, if an interviewer expressed approval of foreign aid (completely unrelated to the subject of the survey) the respondent might infer that the interviewer was in favor of the Tennessee Valley Authority (subject of the survey) because he thought the two opinions were correlated. Whether the respondent is right or wrong in his inference is quite irrelevant; the important thing is that he may modify his response in terms of what he thinks and that this modification results in a biased opinion.

To reduce indirect suggestion as a source of bias, the interviewer must try to make himself as much of a nonentity as possible. In so doing he must not, however, commit the error of trying to hide what he is by assuming different characteristics. This is just as undesirable. He must try to have literally no characteristics. It is, of course, impossible not to have *any* characteristics. The interviewer is, after all, male or female, of a certain age, employed as an interviewer, and the owner of a certain make and model of automobile. These attributes are quite general, how-ever, and probably do not provide very usable clues to respondents. More distinctive clues, and therefore potentially more biasing ones, are dress, language used, opinions expressed, statements of origin, class, and affilia-tions ("I belong to the Elks too, Brother"), and preferences and activities ("I'm a stamp collector myself"). Such information about the interviewer is especially likely to be passed on while rapport is being built, and many interviewers specifically base rapport-building on things they and respondents have in common, or are thought to have in common. *This is a gross error,* for although it is true that respondents are likely to be quite frank and honest with an apparent peer on most questions, there may be some questions on which they have deviant opinions which they will hesitate to reveal to an interviewer precisely *because* he is perceived as a peer. So far as the respondent is concerned the interviewer must not belong to his peer group nor to any other group.

D. *Failure to Discriminate Acceptable from Unacceptable Responses*

The fact that probing is a necessary tool of interviewing implies that not all responses are acceptable. Responses may be incomplete, irrelevant, unclear, inconsistent, lacking in detail, or even false. Excepting false responses, these unacceptable types of responses are fairly easily detected from the responses proper and the knowledge the interviewer has of the respondent and of his previous answers. Completeness, relevancy, and amount of detail given in a response is, of course, a relative matter and must be evaluated against the objectives of questions. *The interviewer must therefore be thoroughly familiar with what information questions are designed to elicit.* Whether responses are clear and meaningful is usually self-evident, but the interviewer must beware of the *meaning* respondents attach to certain words. An extreme example of a word which meant literally one thing but which had an opposite meaning to the respondent occurred recently in a televised interview. The sidewalk respondent was asked what he thought of publicizing the names of juvenile delinquents. He said, "I think it will definitely *curtail* teenage crimes." However, after a few more minutes of questioning it became apparent that *curtail* meant *increase* to the respondent. Actually it it not rare for respondents to use words incorrectly; fortunately these individuals are spotted fairly easily by their conversation, and the interviewer can use clarity probes when the meaning of a word or whole response is suspect.

Wholly or partially false responses are usually difficult to detect and it is believed that good rapport reduces their occurrence to a minimum. Very often a questionnaire will contain several closely related questions such that false responses to one or two of them may be detected from the resulting incongruities. That is, when two or more responses to related questions appear to have a low probability of occurring together the interviewer may rightly suspect the responses and use appropriate probes, even high pressure probes if rapport is sufficiently good. When there is no suggestive evidence that a respondent is prevaricating, but the question is potentially a "sensitive" one, general probing is called for to determine whether the initial response should be accepted. Many times a slight discrepancy with the original response comes to light after probing, and when this discrepancy is used as a basis for further probing the respondent's "true" feelings or opinions will be revealed. The interviewer must take care, however, that the probing in no way endanger the atmosphere of permissiveness.

E. *Failure to Record Responses Adequately*

Although there is no excuse for recording responses inadequately, it is nevertheless done frequently. Recording errors take several forms, but the effect of all is to make data analysis difficult. What is worse, these errors may result in biased estimates of responses.

Common recording errors are incomplete records of responses, distortions of the meaning of responses, the use of abbreviations which are unintelligible to the coder or analyst, illegible handwriting, the failure to record probes and incidents occurring during the interview, the failure to indicate reasons for non-responses, and the recording of the interviewer's own interpretation of responses without identifying these as interpretations. How these errors can be prevented is too obvious to warrant discussion. However, good advice is for the interviewer to place himself in the position of the coder or analyst and then to decide whether his interview records would be meaningful.

Suggested Readings

Hyman, Herbert H., *et al. Interviewing in Social Research.* Chicago: University of Chicago Press, 1954. 415 pp. A somewhat technical discussion of interviewing, interviewer effects and biases, and means of controlling interviewer errors. The interviewer who reads this book will gain much insight into the processes of interviewing.

Kahn, R. L. and C. F. Cannell. *The Dynamics of Interviewing.* New York: John Wiley & Sons, Inc., 1957. A sophisticated, theoretically oriented treatise on the interviewing process viewed as communicative interaction.

Maccoby, Eleanor E. and Nathan Maccoby. "The Interview: A Tool of Social Science," in Gardner Lindzey (ed.), *Handbook of Social Psychology.* Cambridge, Mass.: Addison-Wesley Publishing Company, Inc., 1954. Chapter XII. This is unquestionably the best, most penetrating brief discussion of interviewing available.

Merton, Robert K., Marjorie Fiske, and Patricia L. Kendall. *The Focused Interview: A Manual of Problems and Procedures.* Glencoe, Ill.: Free Press, 1956. 186 pp. Although the discussion in this book is primarily concerned with focused interviews, there is much insight on the practice of probing and other interviewing techniques.

Parten, Mildren B. *Surveys, Polls, and Samples.* New York: Harper & Brothers, 1950. 624 pp. A very extensive, easily read handbook of survey techniques which includes 1,145 references.

Rogers, Carl R. *Counseling and Psychotherapy.* New York: Houghton Mifflin Company, 1942. 420 pp. Although addressed primarily to clinical psychologists and psychiatrists, it should be in the library of every professional interviewer. The concept of nondirective permissive interviewing originated with Rogers and is thoroughly discussed in this book.

Stycos, J. Mayone. *Family and Fertility in Puerto Rico: A Study of the Lower Income Group.* New York: Columbia University Press, 1955. 332 pp. Appendix A, "Methodology," includes a detailed discussion of probing.

Young, Pauline V., *et al. Scientific Social Surveys and Research* (third edition). Englewood Cliffs, N.J.: Prentice-Hall, Inc., 1956. 540 pp. Contains very good discussions of survey designs and techniques with particular emphasis on social surveys. The book is addressed to students of sociology, but, for the most part, can be read easily by any intelligent layman.

Glossary

Action. Technical term used in this manual to denote whether an ODU has been contacted, not contacted, or substituted; or whether an individual has been interviewed, not interviewed, or substituted. The term refers to ODU's and individuals that have been designated for contact and interview.

Area segment. The area of land within which ODU's are sampled. Area segments are usually bounded by easily identified landmarks such as streets, roads, railroad tracks, streams, power lines, etc. The term is usually abbreviated to "segment."

Audimeter. A device used by A. C. Nielson Co. which is installed on a radio or TV set and which records what stations were tuned in, when, and for how long.

Biased. A term describing a response that is not the respondent's true response, or a statistic whose average value does not equal the true value in the universe being sampled.

Call-back. A revisit of the interviewer either to contact an ODU or to interview an individual.

Census. A complete enumeration of a population.

Cruise. To drive around an area segment to locate it unmistakably and to locate dwelling units within it.

Designated. Selected for contact or interview by the sampling procedure.

Dichotomous question. A question which has two specific response alternatives (e.g., "yes" or "no").

Dwelling unit. A group of rooms or a single room occupied by, or intended for occupancy by, one household. It is distinguished from a physical structure (e.g., a house) which may contain one or more dwelling units.

Head of household. The principal "bread winner" in the household, or in some cases the senior male or female in the household, irrespective of his or her economic contribution.

Household. All persons, without regard to relationship, living together with common housekeeping arrangements, including kitchen facilities, in the same dwelling unit. Institutions, commercial rooming houses, fraternities and sororities, military barracks, and transient accommodations and their occupants are not usually regarded as households.

IDS. Abbreviation for ODU Identification Sheet.

Imaginary line. A line or similar demarcation on a map which has no physical counterpart; for example, a county line or a line drawn by the researcher to bound part of an area segment.

Individual. A person in the universe to be sampled. A person technically becomes an individual when he meets the criteria of membership in the universe specified by the researcher.

Individual Identification Sheet (INID). The form on which the interviewer lists all persons living in an ODU and which he uses to designate individuals for sampling.

INID. Abbreviation for Individual Identification Sheet.

Instrument. A device with which specified events, objects, or items of behavior are measured. In surveys the device is usually a question.

Interviewer. The person who obtains interviews and acts as the researcher's agent in that capacity.

Multiple choice question. A question which has more than two specific response alternatives. It is sometimes referred to as a "cafeteria" question.

Occupied dwelling unit (ODU). A dwelling unit which is occupied. It is distinguished from a dwelling unit, which may or may not be occupied.

ODU. Abbreviation for occupied dwelling unit.

ODU Identification Sheet (IDS). The form on which the interviewer lists all ODU's in an area segment and which he uses to designate ODU's for contact.

Open-end. Not providing specific response alternatives, as in open-end questions.

Panel. A sample of respondents interviewed on at least two different occasions. A panel is frequently used in the study of political opinions during major elections, in consumer goods studies, and in audience surveys.

Permissive. Allowing the free expression of any thought, belief, opinion, feeling, or fact.

Probe. A device, usually in the form of a question, used to clarify a response or to obtain additional information from a respondent.

Program Analyzer. A device with two buttons which members of an audience press to indicate whether they like or dislike parts of a program. The "likes" and "dislikes" are recorded on a graph.

Questionnaire. A written collection of questions and instructions relating thereto used to obtain information from respondents.

Random. Having the property of not being predictable beyond chance.

Random number. A number having the property of not being predictable beyond chance. Tables of random numbers are often used in probability sampling.

Rapport. A condition between interviewer and respondent in which the occurrence of complete, unbiased responses is maximized.

Refusal. Unwillingness to be interviewed or otherwise to participate in a survey.

Reliability. The property of an instrument which yields the same measures on repeated occasion. It is usually specified as a fraction or proportion of a theoretical maximum.

Respondent. An individual who gives an interview.

Response. An answer to a question or a reply to a statement relevant to the survey.

Sample (n.). The units (e.g., individuals, ODU's, segments) selected to represent the universe from which they were drawn.

Sample (v.t.). To select a portion of units from a universe of units.

Segment. See *Area segment.*

Segment Sketch Sheet (SSS). The form on which the interviewer makes a sketch of an area segment and locates the dwelling units, ODU's, and sample ODU's within it.

Sensitive question. A question which threatens, embarrasses, or arouses an emotional reaction in the respondent.

SSS. Abbreviation for Segment Sketch Sheet.

Substitution. Contacting an ODU not originally designated for contact when the originally designated ODU could not be contacted, or interviewing an individual not originally designated for interview when the originally designated individual could not be interviewed. Some rules of substitution are given in detail in the text.

Unbiased. A term describing a response that is the respondent's true response, or a statistic whose average equals the true value in the universe being sampled.

Unit. General term referring to a single entity of specified characteristics.

Unit of Observation. The unit (e.g., an individual) upon which measurements are performed.

Universe. The totality of units (e.g., persons, ODU's, area segments) meeting criteria specified by the researcher.

Validity. The property of an instrument which measures what it is intended to measure.

Index